Paleo
For
Beginners

Essential Paleo Diet Cookbook and Guide With 42 Easy Recipes To Get You Started

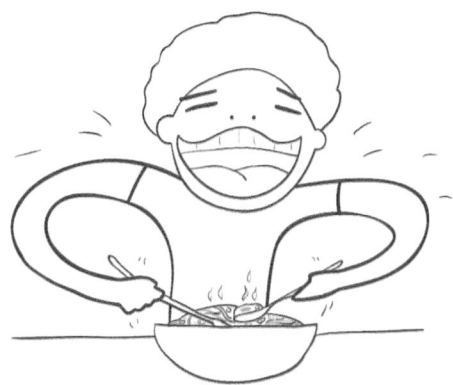

Table of Contents

Basic Recipes to Get You Started

Homemade Ingredients

Breakfast Recipes

Introduction

If you are reading this book, chances are you have some inkling of what the Paleo Diet is.

Maybe you're just curious, maybe you're already sold; either way, you probably have a lot of questions before you're ready to commit to a new lifestyle. And who could blame you?

Diet fads come and go. Some are more substantial than others, some are outright scams designed to help you drop money, not pounds.

The Paleo diet is a relative newcomer, but its roots go back further than any of the new diets you hear about, and it has the power to change your life more deeply than you'd expect.

The purpose of this book is to answer your questions; to help you make an informed decision about the changes you want to make and ease you into a new, healthier lifestyle.

We'll be taking the first steps of your journey with you, so that you feel confident when it's time to walk your own path.
We all needed a parent holding on to the seat of our bike the first time we rode without training wheels.

This book fulfills the same role.

We'll be touching on some of the science and thinking that underlies the Paleo Lifestyle (don't worry, no math!) and we'll go through the transition from a wayward modern diet to a hearty, healthy Paleo diet step by step.

If you follow the guidelines in this book, your Paleo journey will make you feel great about yourself, and get you the results you want.

This isn't a cookbook per se – we'll mostly be focusing on the thought process and beginning steps of the diet – but we have included a choice selection of starter recipes just to get the ball rolling.

These days there are literally thousands of great cookbooks and websites where you can expand your Paleo palate, and no matter what you're craving, somebody out there has made it Paleo.

Once you understand the fundamentals we'll be going over, you're free to roam the world of Paleo recipes unfettered.

We hope you enjoy what we've put together for you, but most of all we hope you can walk away from this book feeling like the champion we know you can be!

So, What Is Paleo Anyway?

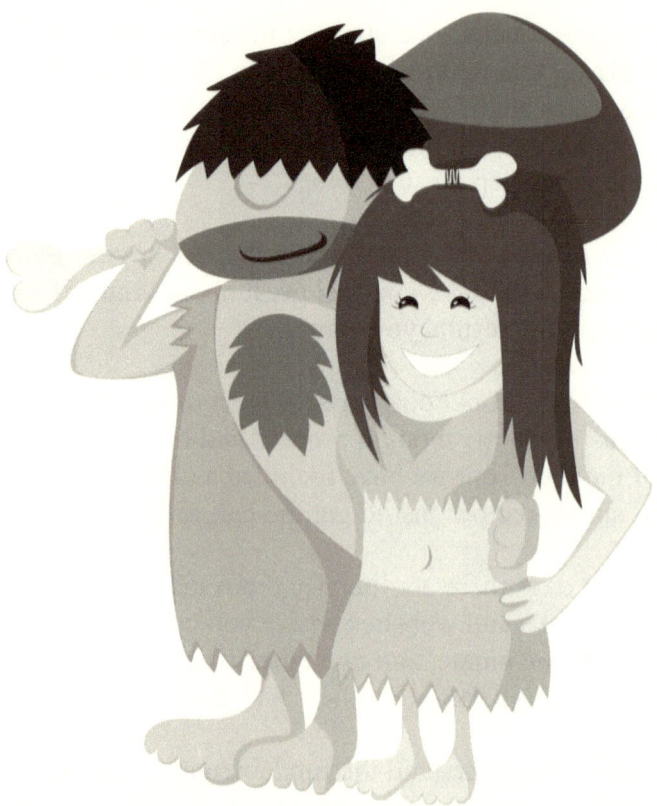

Once upon a time, there was a gentle cave dweller named... oh, let's call him Buk.

Buk was a simple guy with very few things on his mind. Every morning he woke up with the sun, walked out of his cave and went hunting.

Now, Buk happened to live in a temperate forest region, so there were always plenty of deer, boar, birds and squirrels around.

When Buk was a boy, his dad taught him how to make a bow and arrow and how to track and kill the animals that lived in the forest.

So all day, every day, Buk tracked deer, trapped boar, shot ducks and quail, and caught squirrels and other rodents. He skinned them himself, and carried them back to the cave.

Meanwhile, Buk's cavewoman, Wanda, was busy making her rounds in the forest. She dug up roots, plucked berries, climbed trees to fetch fruit and bird eggs, picked mushrooms, and yanked up vegetables. Every night they would get together, roast the spoils of the day over the fire and eat them.

Once upon a very different time, there was a young woman named Jane. Jane worked in an office downtown, had three kids in grade school, and a husband, Jack, who traveled for work.

Every morning, Jane woke before dawn, rustled the kids out of bed, chugged a cup of coffee and piled everybody into the car.

On the way to school, they would drive through the fast food restaurant around the corner and order a bag of greasy styrofoam and cram it down in the car.

After the kids were at school, Jane headed to work, where she usually found a doughnut or bagel lying around in the morning meeting, told herself not to eat it, then ate it anyway.

Around noon, she'd walk down to the corner store and pick up a microwaved burrito and a 44 oz soda.

When she finally got home after spending an hour and a half in traffic, she was too tired to even think about cooking, so she asked Jack to pick up a pizza on the way home from the airport.

The family would chow down, then kick back on the couch with a bag of chips to watch the latest celebrity dance contest on their DVR.

Who do you think was healthier? Buk and Wanda, or Jane and Jack?

The very obvious answer is the entire root of the Paleo Lifestyle. Once upon a time, everyone bore the responsibility of their own food production. The very act of putting together a meal took everyone in the tribe working together. We had to run, jump and climb just to get at the meager scraps that sustained us!

Even more importantly, everything came directly from nature to our bellies. There were no factories to add "cellulose powder" (sawdust!) to our food, and there were no immense farms to pump our chickens and cows full of hormones and antibiotics. A boar was a boar, not a smoked sausage with cheese. A raspberry was a raspberry, not a powdered raspberry-flavor smoothie.

Times were harder, but simpler – and the food was healthier. There were no court cases to try, no TPS reports to write, no math tests to grade, all we had to do was eat, build shelters, and socialize with each other.

But the world is different now, and it's not going to change back. Unless you're Chuck Norris, you probably aren't tough enough to go completely off the grid and live like Buk and Wanda. And unless you're a survivalist, you probably don't want to. We like our cell phones. We like our first-person-shooter video games, our DVRs, our microwaves and hamburgers. So how do we bring together the best of the past and the best of now?

The Paleo lifestyle. With just a few simple ideas, and a small amount of prep-work, you can have it both ways. Thankfully, good food still exists, and there is a growing trend towards eating cleaner. It's not only better for our bodies, but it's better for the planet.

Choosing responsibly produced and sourced food will keep mysterious chemicals out of your diet, and help support the farmers and ranchers that want to keep them out of the environment.

What the Paleo lifestyle attempts to do is guide us towards eating the things our bodies were made to eat. Early humans adapted to eating the spoils of their environment only. Their tummies weren't exposed to the processed science experiments we call food these days. And our bodies have changed very little, if at all, since those days. The change in our diet has *massively* outpaced the change in how our bodies process food.

The Paleo approach attempts to put our bodies and our food back in sync.

You wouldn't put diesel fuel in your gas car, would you? Your car wouldn't be able to use it. You might get a sputter or a spark here and there, but the car's engine definitely wouldn't run right.

Your body is no different.

By fueling it with things that it isn't meant to consume, you're ensuring that it won't run properly. But if you start fueling it the way it was built to be fueled, it'll run the way it was built to run.

You have the potential to be as strong and vital as Buk and Wanda. You can climb, run, and jump all day, once you have your body running right.

All you have to do is get back on track.

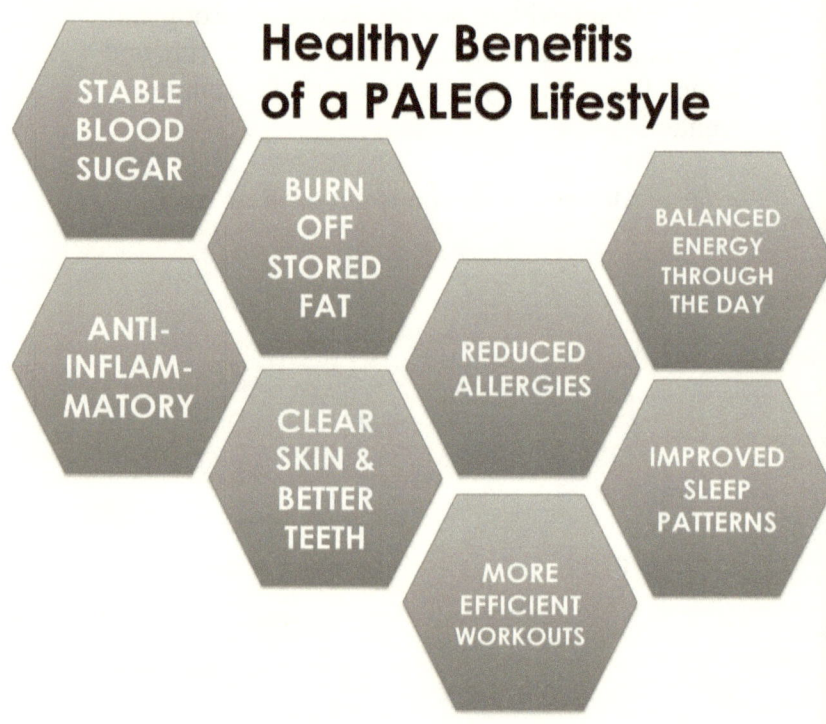

Healthy Benefits
of a PALEO Lifestyle

STABLE BLOOD SUGAR

BURN OFF STORED FAT

BALANCED ENERGY THROUGH THE DAY

ANTI-INFLAM-MATORY

REDUCED ALLERGIES

CLEAR SKIN & BETTER TEETH

IMPROVED SLEEP PATTERNS

MORE EFFICIENT WORKOUTS

Natural Weight Loss with the Paleo Lifestyle

The Paleo Lifestyle is exactly that – a lifestyle. It goes well beyond a simple diet plan. Rather, it strives to be a set of guiding principles that will put your body back in sync with its original design.

We all know how weight loss and gain works. You eat more than you need to, and the extra is stored as fat. You eat less, and your body will start to burn that excess fat to make up the difference. Your body is going to get it's daily quota of energy however it can.

One issue that has only recently come to light, however, is that what gets stored as fat is not only determined by *how much* is eaten, but by *what* is eaten.

Your body knows exactly what to do with an apple. It metabolizes the natural sugars into the bloodstream and sends it to your muscles and organs, where it is burned for energy. Your stomach then sends the fiber down into your lower digestive organs and it aids in passing your waste.

On the other hand, your body doesn't have a clue what to do with a chicken nugget. Some of it is protein, sure, and there are some carbohydrates there that can be turned into energy, but what about all that MSG? TBHQ?

That stuff gets lost in your organs, searching for a home.

And what about all that hydrogenated fat? It's no use to your body, and besides, there's more of it than your body knows what to do with at any given moment. So most of it ends up in your fat cells, put away until your body can figure out what to do about it.

And fat and carbs together? That's about the most confusing combination your body can get.

It sends your blood sugar into a fit that wrecks you body's ability to regulate hunger. That way, you to keep going back for that next chicken nugget, and before you know what's happening you've eaten 40 of them. You then sink into a blood sugar slump where you feel tired and bloated. The food you've eaten – which was supposed to give you energy – has had the exact opposite of the desired effect!

Losing Weight with the Paleo Diet

The way your body can lose weight with the Paleo diet is twofold:

First, you stop feeding your body things it doesn't know how to handle.

This keeps them out of your organs, bloodstream and fat cells.

Second, you reduce your intake of carbohydrates to the point where your body switches over to burning fat as its primary energy source.

This state is called Ketosis, and it is the heart of weight loss with the Paleo Lifestyle.

When your body is burning fat as it's primary fuel, it changes the way your body processes fat when you eat. Without a significant amount of carbs to burn, it burns the fat first. Luckily for us, fat is a much less energy-efficient fuel than carbs. Carbs burn like wax; slow and steady, with very little energy. Fat burns like rocket fuel; fast, energetic, but not long-lasting. Your body will burn up the fat quicker, causing it to dip into its fat reserves sooner. That way, when you exercise, you'll be getting more bang for your buck.

If you keep active (remember, Buk was running around a forest *all day*) you'll be dipping into these reserves often.

You don't have to work as hard as Buk did (after all, you've got a life), but a little a day will produce bigger results when your body is running on fat.

Once you're getting closer to your ideal weight, you can begin phasing in those higher-carb foods that still fit in with the Paleo Lifestyle.

If you're going for weight loss, you won't want to incorporate things like sweet potatoes to your diet at first, but once you're at your goal they won't pack the pounds back on either. The carb-heavy foods tolerated by the Paleo Lifestyle are healthier and more natural than the type we're used to eating in today's society, and your body will handle them better once you've reached your weight loss goal. Especially if you keep active.

The best recommendation as far as activity goes is to keep it fun and natural. After a few weeks, the treadmill can start to feel like a chore.

Not only that, but it's hardly stimulating for the mind. The best activities are self-encouraging – you won't have to force yourself to do them.

Take up a sport like basketball or tennis. Even if you can't afford country-club dues, or can't get a team to shoot hoops, a few minutes a day bouncing a ball off the garage door is more fun than a Stairmaster.

Try taking a brisk walk around the neighborhood or the local park. You might even find a little hidden adventure every now and then. Don't be afraid to wander.

These types of activities are great because they're fun for their own sake, not just as exercise.

It's far better to feel like you're doing something fun and just *happen* to be exercising while you do it. That's the way it was in Buk's day, and that's the way it should be for you.

At your ideal weight, and fueled by a clean diet, you'll be running at peak performance, just like Buk was. And you won't need any fancy pills or powdered shakes to do it. Just good, simple, clean eating and a taste for fun, rewarding exercise.

That's why we call it natural weight loss. It's not a scientifically designed system. It's simple; it's just your life, and if you do it this way, it'll be a good one.

Improved Health with the Paleo Lifestyle

The reason we hesitate to call this approach a "diet" is because the idea of a diet carries with it a connotation of temporariness.

People go on diets, lose weight and then go off them. And after decades of hearing the news stories, testimonials and debunking rants, we know that a temporary diet is nearly always a bad solution to our health problems. It treats our weight and basic health like a disease, we cure it, then move on.

But your health isn't like that. Your health is an evolving state that you always carry with you. You can't treat it temporarily if you're unsatisfied with it.

You have to make permanent changes.

So Paleo requires some commitment. You have to be willing to stick to these ideals for life. The reward is that if you do, you will slowly watch your body transform into something better than it was before.

In a very basic way, the human body is *made entirely* of food. Your hair is made of proteins and minerals. Your skin moisturizes itself with oils – fats. Your blood carries various types of sugars. Your organs process and break down various kinds of vitamins and minerals. Your bones are made of minerals.

Every seven years, your body is completely new. Some cell turnover is rapid, some gradual, but over the course of your life, you will be made of completely different molecules than the ones you were born with.

And the ones you were born with? That's right, your parents' bodies built them out of food. We *literally* are what we eat.

So why eat things that the human body wasn't meant to use as building blocks? When we do that, we end up with inflamed cells, overtaxed and poisoned organs, excess fat, chronic disease, cell mutation (cancer) and total systematic breakdown. The unnatural compounds we eat are literally unmaking our bodies on a molecular level.

But our bodies are efficient. They have the power to remake themselves, and they do it in spite of us.

If we stop introducing harmful substances into them, the existing harmful substances will eventually be gone. Some systems in our bodies will take a while to renew themselves, but it is literally never too late to start.

We could quote you a bunch of studies, but that isn't what this book is about. This book is about conveying basic principles. If you want the hard data, it is widely available on the internet (if we recounted it all here, you'd probably want to check our story out anyway!)

We're all smart enough to know that our cells are constantly remaking themselves, and they can only use the building blocks we provide to achieve that. If we provide them better materials, and less foreign contaminants, our bodies will eventually clean themselves out and start working the way they are meant to.

We don't need to read you the riot act. You're smart enough to see the obvious reasons why this approach works.

You might still have a little to learn when it comes to understanding which foods are clean and which aren't, but that's another chapter.

Cleaning Out the Pantry – Time to Commit!

This part of the process might be a little scary.

Grab yourself a clean garbage bag or other large container, and begin clearing your pantry of everything that isn't Paleo.

What is and isn't Paleo, you ask? We'll be getting more specific later on, but for now, we're mainly concerned with anything that isn't 100% straight from nature. That means pretty much anything with a label, unfortunately.

That might be most of your food, but that's why we suggest taking everything you get rid of down to your local church or homeless shelter and donating it. If it's sealed, they'll take it. If not, you and they are better off without it.

If it's got nutrition facts and a label, you're going to want to get rid of it. If it's an all-natural product, read the ingredients list. Anything you do not know to be plant or animal-derived? Anything you can't pronounce, or anything that has (parentheses) next to it? Toss it.

This initial purge is going to make sure you aren't tempted by a stray box of wheat crackers or chocolate chip cookies. If it's out of your house, it can't hurt you.

All carbohydrate products must go. In the beginning stages of the Paleo Lifestyle it's best to err on the side of caution with carbs, especially if you're in it for weight loss. Carbs (especially those filled with artificial chemicals) mess with your blood sugar regulation and cause you to develop unhealthy eating habits.

Your body is hard-wired to desire carbs – they are by far the most efficient source of food-energy. But you're going to be reprogramming your body, so they have to go. This means cereal, bread, flour, pastries, pasta, rice, couscous, beans, lentils, oatmeal, cornmeal, grits, cream of wheat, anything you would serve as a starch or use to make something starchy.

This is also a good time to talk about legumes. Generally, legumes are fruits that grow in pods of two or more.

The problem with legumes is that they are actually packed with toxins, even in their 100% natural state. They are also often laden with carbs that digest poorly, as well as high concentrations of fat that make it harder to regulate your intake.

So peanuts, beans, green peas, chickpeas (hummus!), lentils, all of them have to go.

The only exception to this rule is green beans, which can be consumed raw, and digest more like a vegetable. They also contain only trace amounts of the toxins present in many legumes, so they are generally regarded as a safe part of a Paleo lifestyle.

There's a bit of debate around the subject of dairy products on the Paleo diet. On the one hand, many dairy products are produced in factory settings that pump them full of unhealthy additives.

Additionally, paleolithic humans like Buk and Wanda didn't milk cows or make sour cream. But on the other hand, our own mothers breast-fed us the milk that their bodies produced. The nutrients included everything we needed to survive those early years, and it was in fact the healthiest thing for us at that stage in our life.

Our bodies are made – arguably – to process at least *some* dairy products.

The devil, however is in the details. If you have a readily available supply of all natural, raw dairy products (a growing trend), then by all means include them in your diet. If not, you might be better off without dairy, at least at first.

The real trick is to test your body and see what it tolerates. Try going without it for two weeks. If you notice an improvement, good. Then add it back in. If you still feel great, super.

If you notice that you feel sluggish, or bloated, or have any digestive issues, then cut it out for good. But at first, it's probably a good idea to steer clear of all dairy products, just to get a fresh start.

That means milk, cheese, yogurt, sour cream, coffee creamer, all of it has to go. If you have real butter, go ahead and keep that, though. Later, we'll cover a recipe that allows you to convert it into a healthy Paleo ingredient called ghee.

On to sweets. Anything that you would consider a sweet treat has to go. Any artificial sweeteners too. Like starchy products, sweets are loaded with carbohydrates, only they're simple, so-called "fast" carbs, that burn up in an instant and cause cravings for more.

Processed sugar is the cocaine of the carbohydrate world; it makes you feel great for a short burst of time and then you crash hard. All the while, it's wreaking havoc on your body, causing it to substitute your body's innate chemicals for this new, hyper-powered substance.

Eventually, your body can stop producing those chemicals and you wind up with diabetes.

To put it plainly, processed sugars are bad news, and they all need to go, even if you aren't going Paleo. We would all be better off without them. That means cookies, candy, baked goods, pastries, white and brown sugar, sugar substitutes, syrup, honey, sweetened coffee creamers, sugared breath mints, diet and regular sodas, sports drinks, pre-made smoothies and shakes, all of it must be disposed of.

Caffeine products are the next step.

We know many people feel they can't function without caffeine; now is the time to overcome that illusion. Chances are that part of the reason you feel this way is because you are feeding yourself an unbalanced diet of foods that provide shoddy, unhealthy energy.

Your blood sugar isn't properly regulated, so you get tired. Caffeine fills the gaps. But our bodies are made to derive their energy from food, and that is the direction you are going to be moving in.

So dump the coffee, toss the strong black teas, and ditch the caffeinated sodas.

You're bound to go through a little withdrawal, but hey, no pain, no gain. You will get through it, we promise. Caffeine can also trigger carb cravings, which will make it much harder to stick to your new, clean regime. So even if it hurts, you must rid yourself of it, at least at first.

Alcohol needs to go too. Because alcohol is often quite expensive, and because the homeless shelter is unlikely to take it, we wouldn't actually suggest throwing it all away.

Rather, you might want to stash it all in an inconvenient location; say the basement or the garage. Somewhere it won't spoil (if you're a wine or beer drinker), but somewhere that it won't be in your face every time you get thirsty.

Get it out of the fridge, at least. You aren't likely to be tempted by warm beer or chardonnay. If you can keep alcohol out of your sight, that should be good enough.

And if the idea of not drinking for a few weeks scares you, you might need more than a change in diet.

Alcohol, even consumed in moderation, makes it difficult for your body to function, and darn near impossible to lose weight.

Alcohol digests similarly to sugar carbs (many alcoholic products contain sugar and complex carbs as well), and has a similar effect on your blood sugar.

It also decreases inhibition, which can make it easier to make poor food decisions. Who among us hasn't ended a night on the town by hitting the 24-hour burger joint, or ordering a pizza and scarfing down the whole thing?

In the beginning stages of your Paleo Journey, you're better off without the stuff, especially if you're trying to drop a few pounds.

That means beer, wine, liquor, sweetened cordials, all of it must go.

Now that you've cleaned everything out, your fridge and pantry probably look pretty bare!

This might scare you a bit, but in the next chapters we'll be going over how to fill it back up again, and this time, we'll be filling it up healthy and natural.

Shopping – General Tips

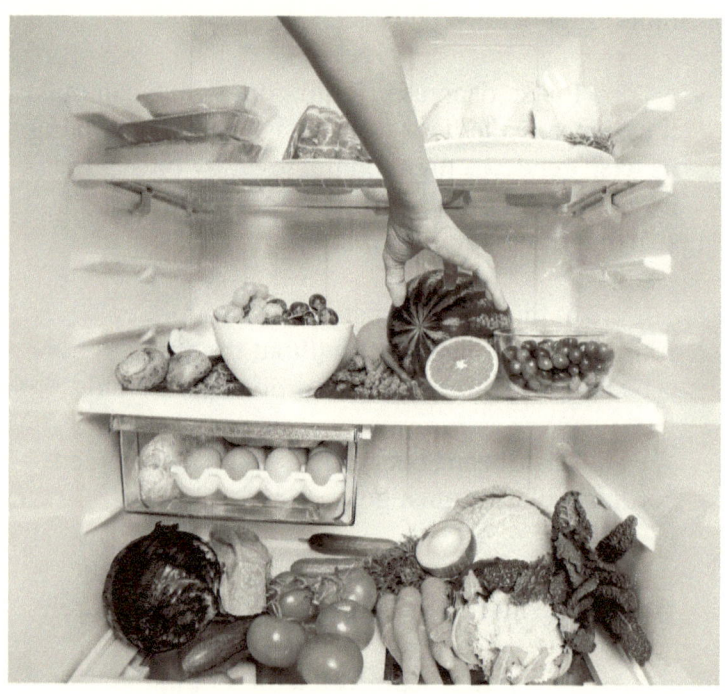

After the last chapter, you probably have a pretty good idea of what's forbidden on the Paleo diet. If not, don't worry, more specifics are coming, in an easy-to-reference list. For now, however, we're going to focus on how to navigate the grocery store like a caveman.

If we didn't know any better, we'd say the grocery store was set up to trick you into getting fat. Everywhere you look there are big shiny displays of sugary, processed foods, salty snacks and convenient prepared foods. It's easy to be drawn into buying whatever the store owners want you to buy.

The truth is that the store's number one goal is to make money, not make you healthy. Even if you're shopping local, or at a natural food store, cash is the bottom line. So the stores are designed to direct you to the thing which make the owners the most money, which are nearly always things that are cheap to produce.

The food companies cut corners and substitute artificial chemicals for more expensive natural products, and they pass the savings to the grocery store. The grocery store then marks them up, puts them right out front in a loud display (or at eye level on the shelf), and they reap the maximum profit margin.

This means you need to walk into the grocery store with a plan – and stick to it. Without a list, or at least a general plan of attack, you're bound to be sucked in to buying whatever the store wants to sell you.

Luckily, you can avoid much of the bad stuff with one simple rule: shop the outside edges of the store, and steer clear of the center aisles. The edges of the store include departments like produce, dairy, meat and seafood. Often the freezer aisles will be arranged closer to the edges of the store, and there is a lot of Paleo goodness in there too.

Another good bit of advice is: don't go to the store hungry! If you're starving while you shop, your resolve will be much lower, and you'll be tempted to do something rash. When you're full, your brain is working right, and you'll have a much easier time making sound decisions.

Products have labels. Products can be easily shelved, and have a long shelf life. Food, on the other hand, rarely comes with a label, brand or box. Food spoils faster, and so it needs refrigeration, or even freezing. Food is hard to stack on a shelf in a pretty little line; food needs to be kept in a big pile.

Maybe this doesn't sound so flattering, but the reality is that food is beautiful. Fruits and vegetables come in all kinds of vibrant colors. Fresh meats have deep, rich color, and you can even smell the savory flavor they carry. Real food assaults the senses with the promise of deliciousness and nutrition.

Products look and smell like cardboard. When you have a cart full of real food, things which are recognizable to the eye and free from mystery, there is no better feeling.

For many people, this is the turning point in their Paleo journey, the moment when they start becoming proud of the choices they are making.

So eat a good meal before you go to the store, and shop the edges. Stick to produce, responsibly raised meats, fresh (and preferably raw) dairy and simple frozen ingredients like vegetables.

Chances are you'll look down at the cart and smile every time.

Foods to Eat and Avoid – Specific Tips

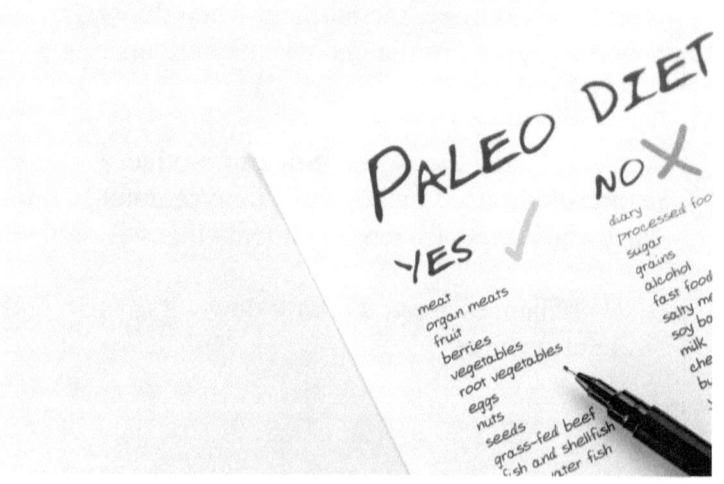

Now we get down to the nitty gritty.

In this chapter we're going to go through some items category-by-category so you'll have a greater understanding of what to do at the grocery store.

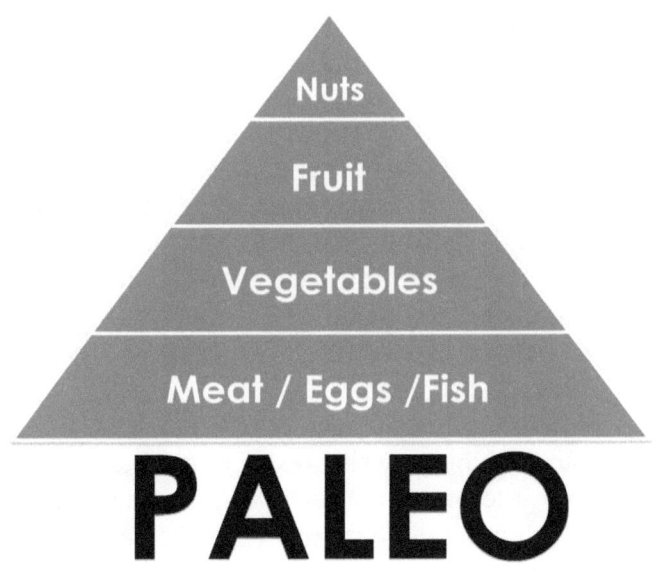

Meats:

The main thing with meats is that you want something that is responsibly raised.

That means all-natural, cruelty-free if possible, and never any hormones, steroids or other sketchy additives. When it comes to land creatures (beef, pork, chicken, and game), you want grass-fed, or pastured.

This means the animal grew up on a healthy diet consisting mainly of the things *its* body was designed to eat. It's essentially passing the health along to you; the animal was eating Paleo, so you are.

Factory-farmed meat is full of chemicals that can cause all sorts of problems, not the least of which is cellular inflammation. Your entire body can be negatively impacted, from your immune system to your nervous system. So stick to anything that carries a sticker saying "grass-fed" "all-natural" or "pastured".

Game meats are also great. These are a little harder to find, but any self-respecting butcher shop will have at least a small selection. Game animals live in their natural environment, so they eat their natural diet.

If you *must* but factory farmed meat, make sure it is as lean as possible, and stay away from organ meats. Animal bodies work similarly to humans when it comes to artificial chemicals. Anything the animal's body doesn't know how to handle ends up in fat deposits and organs. A well-marbled ribeye that came from a factory-raised cow will have many times more toxins than a sirloin or filet from the same cow.

With seafood, the key is "wild-caught". Wild-caught seafood doesn't have all the extra nastiness that farm-raised seafood carries with it. Like game, these animals feed on their natural diet because they still live in their natural environment. Fresh is best, in terms of quality, but frozen is fine too if it's wild.

And just to make sure you're having the best possible impact on the earth, try not to buy things that are subject to over-fishing. Tuna and any whitefish are chiefest among these. If you have a natural food store nearby, the fish offered there are a much safer bet.

The catch to all this is that you will probably be paying a bit more for your meat. Don't stress about this, it's worth it to get the body and life you want; the body and life you were born to have.

The other silver lining is that this will force you to portion your meat conservatively, and you will develop a habit of proper portioning.

As you progress, you'll find that you didn't need to be eating the amounts you were before, you had just tricked your brain into expecting them, and your blood sugar roller-coaster was making you crave more, even when most of your body knew it had had enough.

So stick to natural, responsibly raised meats. They're tastier, and bound to have a positive impact on your entire diet. If you stick to this, no meat is forbidden.

Feel free to dine on:

- Beef
- Chicken
- Quail
- Duck
- Turkey
- Pork
- Elk
- Venison
- Boar
- Salmon
- Fresh Tuna
- Swordfish
- Crab
- Shrimp
- Octopus
- And much, much more.

Produce:

When it comes to produce, it's all about knowing when to go organic.

Anything that has a natural casing (or that is peeled before eating) can be eaten without regard to whether it's organic. Bananas, citrus (oranges, limes, lemons), avocados, melons, root veggies with inedible peels (jicama, celery root), onions, sweet potatoes, pineapple, coconut, nuts in the shell, firm squash (butternut, acorn, pumpkin), all of these things can be eaten freely.

Most other vegetables, however, should be organic, and if you have a good organic produce market, it can't hurt to go organic all the way. Lettuce, cabbage, zucchini, celery, carrots, apples, berries, herbs, green beans, mushrooms, all these things are best organic.

The good news is that organic produce doesn't cost a whole lot more than the regular stuff, on the whole. It can even be cheaper, if you have a good farmer's market nearby.

One issue that may irritate you is the exclusion of the white potato from the Paleo lifestyle.

"But, they're natural!" you cry in desperation.

The problem with potatoes is that they evolved symbiotically with human agriculture. We have bred them to be almost 100% starch, and very little else. They contain negligible amounts of nutrients, and the carbs contained within them act on your body much like those derived from grains. You just don't get a lot of nutrient bang for your calorie buck, so they just aren't much good to a Paleo Lifestyle.

The good news is that anything a potato can do, some other root veggie can do better. Baked potatoes can be baked sweet potatoes, and even go well with all the same toppings (and many more).

Fried potato dishes can be made from carrots, parsnips and even squash (we have a great recipe in this book, in fact!).

Mashed potatoes can be imitated with a puree of nearly any root vegetable (turnips are nice and neutral, parsnips are naturally sweet and hearty) or even made with pureed cauliflower.

Just imagine the potato dish you want, and there is another veggie that can do it with more flavor and nutrition, ten times out of ten. Just be sure to keep starchy sides to a minimum if you're trying to lose weight.

So stick to the above principles and dine freely on:

- Apples
- Grapes
- Oranges
- Grapefruit
- Lemons
- Limes
- Melons
- Kiwi
- Strawberries
- Blackberries
- Blueberries
- Raspberries
- Plums
- Pears
- Peaches
- Nectarines

- Apricots
- Avocados
- Pineapple
- Banana
- Coconut
- Lettuce
- Greens (Turnip, Beet, Mustard, Collard, etc.)
- Kale
- Cabbage
- Cucumbers
- Celery
- Carrots
- Turnips
- Rutabegas
- Parsnips
- Broccoli
- Cauliflower
- Peppers (Bell, Jalapeno, Ancho, Poblano, etc.)

- Garlic
- Onions
- Mushrooms
- Fresh Herbs (Parsley, Cilantro, Mint, Basil, etc.)
- And much, much more.

Dairy:

As we've already mentioned, dairy is a bit of a gray area.

For weight loss and general health purposes, we recommend you go without for at least two weeks, and then include it only if your energy level and digestive functioning is unaffected.

If you tolerate dairy, make sure it's 100% natural and raw, if possible.

- Raw Milk

- Heavy Cream

- Yogurt that isn't sweetened with sugar

- Butter (clarified, if possible)

- Cheese (fresh is best: ricotta, cottage, mascarpone)

- Sour Cream

- Make sure to real all labels carefully. Anything unusual, any sweeteners or preservatives, and you shouldn't eat it.

Tree Nuts:

Tree nuts can be a great source of protein and healthy fats. But what's the difference between a tree nut, a legume, a seed and a drupe?

Tree nuts contain a single seed in a shell. Legumes contain two or more seeds in a pod. Seeds often come from a flower, or are contained in a fruit. Drupes contain a seed encased in a husk, and either the seed or the husk may be the edible part. The coconut and the almond are both drupes with inedible husks. Peaches and other stonefruit are technically drupes, with edible husks and inedible seeds.

You don't want too much of any of them, however, because the distribution of fats is less than ideal for a high-functioning body.

Legumes are all out: peanuts, beans, green peas, lentils, etc.

As long as they are consumed in moderation, tree nuts, seeds and drupes are in:

- Almonds

- Cashews

- Macadamias

- Pecans

- Walnuts

- Brazil Nuts

- Sesame Seeds

- Sunflower Seeds (in moderation)

- Almond Flour/Meal, and other nut flours

- And more

Oils:

The main issue with oils is that you want them to be derived from products you can eat on the Paleo diet. Corn and other grain-derived oils are out.

Vegetable oil, despite its name, is out because of its poor combination of fats. Soybean, nut and some seed oils are out for the same reason

You want cold-pressed, all natural oils. The best ones are:

– Extra-Virgin Olive Oil

– Grapeseed Oil

– Coconut Oil

Grapeseed and Coconut are ideal for cooking due to their high smoke-point and mild flavor. Olive oil is best used raw, in salad dressings or as a finishing element.

The Coconut Family of Products:

Coconuts and coconut trees have been adapted into a wide range of products that are actually great substitutes for other forbidden products.

– Coconut Oil, as mentioned above

– Coconut Aminos, a great soy sauce substitute

– Coconut Milk, used in cooking in place of milk

– Coconut Flour, as a baking ingredient

Other Products:

There are *some* products that you might find in the center aisles of the store that are actually okay on the Paleo diet.

As with all things, make sure to read the label carefully and avoid any products that contain any chemicals or additives.

- Pickles, so long as they are cold-brined
- Saurkraut, all natural
- Mustard, though it's better to make your own (we have a recipe coming up!)
- Spices and Dried Herbs (but *not* spice mixes, as they often contain too much salt, sugar or other bad things)
- Salt, in moderation
- *Raw*, Unprocessed Honey, in great moderation
- Tea, as long as it is low-caffeine/caffeine-free and organic
- Bottled Water

- Almond Milk, all-natural, additive free (but it's best homemade)
- Tapioca Flour, a root derived flour that functions similar to corn starch in recipes (but much better in your body) and can be used as a thickening agent or a baking ingredient.

- Extremely Dark Chocolate (Chocolate that is 80% cacao or more contains only trace amounts of sugar and usually no dairy products)

- Wine: Wine making goes back almost to Buk's time; it more or less happens in nature due to natural fermentation. Wine should be consumed in great moderation, but an occasional glass won't hurt, after you've acclimated yourself to the diet. We suggest going at least two weeks without.

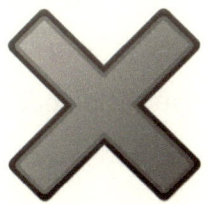

Forbidden Foods:

Some things, however, are definitely out. The foods listed below are to be avoided at all times.

1. All wheat products: bread, flour, crackers, cookies, cereals, pasta, etc.

2. All grains and grain products: corn, cornmeal, cornstarch, corn oil, corn syrup, barley, oats, granola, cereal, rice, rice pudding, rice snacks, etc.

3. Legumes: beans, lentils, peanuts, green peas,etc.

4. Soybeans and *all* soy products! - soy sauce, soy flour, edamame, imitation meats made from soy, etc.

5. All processed sugars and sweeteners: white sugar, brown sugar, molasses, all syrup, agave, Splenda®, Equal®, Sweet and Low®, processed honey, etc.

6. Sweets: candy, ice cream and ice cream treats, even sugar-free

7. Processed meat products: commercial packaged jerky, meat sticks, deli meat containing nitrates or other additives, hot dogs, cured sausages, cured bacon (uncured is becoming more widely available), sugar-cured ham, canned meats, etc. Read all labels carefully!

8. Canned products that contain added salt, sugar or other chemicals

9. Frozen vegetables with sauce

10. Frozen dinners, pizzas or sandwiches

11. Processed cheese products like Velveeta®, or spray-cheese

12. Commercial salad dressings, dips, sauces, condiments and marinades

13. Powdered sauce mixes and packets

14. Powdered drinks

15. Sodas, coffee, caffeinated tea, sweetened juices, basically any drink besides water and homemade beverages.

16. Alcohol, except wine in great moderation

And that's about the long and short of it! With everything, make sure you read any labeling *very carefully!* A lot of seemingly natural products will sneak funky things in there that you are better off without.

Be wary of anything in a cardboard box or plastic bag.

And always, if in doubt, count it out!

The 80/20 Rule

Here's the part where we recognize reality.

We don't live in a perfect world.

What you eat and when you eat is not solely determined by your dietary preferences. And how often have you heard the phrase that if you want to make God laugh, tell him your plans?

The simple truth is that you are going to run into difficulty out there.

Try as you might to eat like Buk, sometimes you are going to encounter a situation where you feel pressure to eat like a modern human.

And that's where the 80/20 rule comes in.

□

The 80/20 Rule:

So long as you're eating clean and Paleo 80% of the time, you will see the benefits.

This doesn't mean you count down the meals/days until you can splurge – and then eat seven meals at drive-thru restaurants.

You don't want your life to revolve around the 20%.

You don't want to view the 20% as a "reward" for good behavior. Better health and a fitter body are the reward for good behavior.

But it's not good to beat yourself up about mistakes either. If you go to a friend's house for dinner and they make mashed potatoes, a small helping won't break your lifestyle apart.

It might be considered rude not to eat something that someone offers you, and acquiescing to the social aspect of eating is not a crime. If you're on a road trip, Paleo food might be hard to find. Sometimes necessity dictates our choices.

When it comes to cravings for specific treats, however, it is recommended that you try to find a Paleo version of that treat.

If you're craving cake, you might try your hand at almond flour muffins.

If you're dying for a scoop of ice cream, see if a little frozen coconut milk with mixed berries and a little dark chocolate doesn't fit the bill.

That's the reason these Paleo imitations exist, to quench the cravings.

But make no mistake, it's still definitely part of your 20%. If you fill your entire diet with these types of items, you're really doing yourself a disservice. Rather than learning to enjoy whole, natural foods for their own sake, you'll be lamenting the fact that you must eat pale imitations of the junk food you crave.

You might technically stay Paleo, but you'll be cheating yourself out of the joy of simple, natural food. You'll also be setting yourself up to fail by keeping your mind focused on the foods you miss, elevating it to an almost mythical status.

This gives the food power over you, and we're looking to have power over our food, just like Buk did.

So use your 20%, but use it wisely. Use it to be polite, use it to calm cravings with a healthy approximation, and use it to keep yourself sane.

The ultimate goal is to improve your life, and if you are constantly beating yourself up, or feeling deprived, then your life may not feel better, even if your diet is.

If you use the 80/20 rule wisely, you will feel like the master of your food.

Meal Plan and Grocery List

Here we've included a sample meal plan just to get your thinking started.

This meal plan keeps it pretty low-carb and 100% dairy-free, as we recommend you stay low-carb and dairy-free at the beginning of your journey.

We've also included a grocery list so you can see how a typical week might stack up. (For simplicity, we'll assume you have a well-stocked spice cabinet)

Monday:

Breakfast: 3 scrambled eggs with mushrooms and green onions; 2 strips of uncured bacon; sliced strawberries

Lunch: grilled marinated chicken breast; steamed broccoli with olive oil; side salad with homemade vinaigrette

Snack: 1/4 cup of roasted almonds; apple

Dinner: mustard-marinated pork chop topped with sauteed onions; grilled zucchini spears; side salad with homemade vinaigrette

---

Tuesday:

Breakfast: 3 fried eggs; parsnip hash

Lunch: chicken salad with grapes and almonds; romaine lettuce; orange

Snack: homemade jerky

Dinner: pan-seared tritip steak; sauteed kale; cucumber and tomato salad with oil, vinegar and herbs

---

Wednesday:

Breakfast: leftover tritip; 2 fried eggs; grapefruit

Lunch: lettuce-wrapped burger with uncured bacon, mustard and mayo; steamed green beans

Snack: banana

Dinner: pollo asada; sauteed onions, mushrooms and peppers; avocado; homemade salsa

---

Thursday:

Breakfast: 3 scrambled eggs with leftover peppers, onions and mushrooms; apple

Lunch: tuna tartare with cucumbers for dipping; broccoli and carrot salad

Snack: carrots; celery with almond butter

Dinner: grilled lamb; parsnip puree; side salad with homemade vinaigrette

---

Friday:

Breakfast: 2 thinly-sliced pork chops topped with grilled onions; orange

Lunch: BBQ marinated chicken; homemade coleslaw; apple

Snack: 1/4 cup roasted almonds; carrots

Dinner: broiled grass-fed ribeye; baked sweet potato with ghee and cinnamon; steamed green beans

---

Saturday:

Breakfast: fritatta with homemade sausage, sauteed mushrooms and kale

Lunch: Asian chicken lettuce wraps with leftover coleslaw; steamed green beans with coconut aminos; orange

Snack: Leftover fritatta

Dinner: seared tuna steak with coconut aminos; stir-fried peppers, onions, mushrooms, carrots and cabbage

---

Sunday:

Breakfast: tapioca flour crepes with warm strawberries; 3 strips uncured bacon

Lunch: grilled chicken breast over romaine lettuce with homemade vinaigrette

Snack: apple, celery with almond butter

Dinner: whole roasted chicken; steamed broccoli; roasted butternut squash

---

Grocery List:

Meats
1. uncured bacon
2. 6 chicken breasts
3. 1 small chicken
4. 2 pork chops
5. 6-8 oz lean grass-fed sirloin (for jerky)
6. 12-16 oz grass-fed tritip steaks
7. 12-16 oz grass-fed ribeye
8. 1/3 lb grass-fed ground beef
9. 8-10 oz fresh tuna steak
10. 4 oz ground pork
11. 24 eggs

Produce
- strawberries
- broccoli
- mushrooms
- green onions
- romaine lettuce
- apples
- oranges
- onions
- zucchini
- parsnips
- grapes
- kale
- cucumbers
- tomatoes

- green beans
- banana
- bell peppers
- avocado
- jalapenos
- cilantro
- fresh herbs
- broccoli
- carrots
- celery
- cabbage
- sweet potato
- butternut squash
- lemons
- limes

Other
- coconut aminos
- olive oil
- grapeseed oil
- vinegar (apple cider, balsamic, white or red wine)
- spices (as needed)
- almonds
- almond butter
- tapioca flour
- ground mustard
- butter (to make ghee)

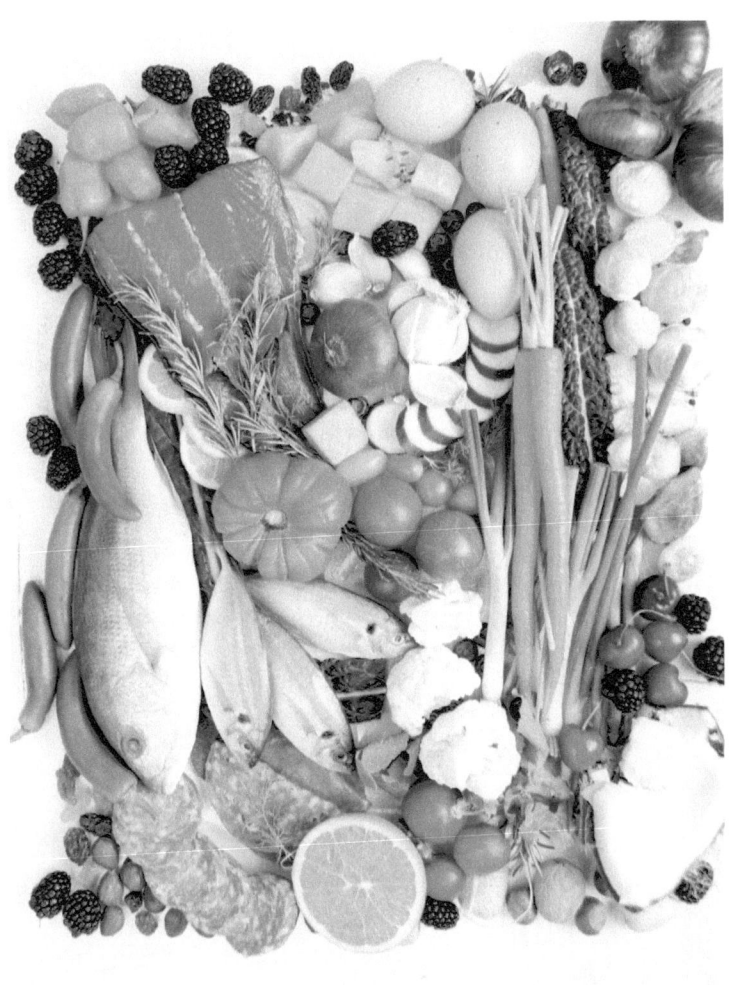

Basic Recipes to Get You Started

Here is a collection of foundational recipes that you can build on to create a unique Paleo menu.

Everything here is presented in its simplest form; that way it's open to interpretation and invention.

When you've mastered the recipes in this book, you'll be ready to walk into the wide world of Paleo cooking. There are literally thousands of websites, boasting millions of recipes for you to try.

The Paleo Lifestyle isn't about limits.

It's about reprogramming our food and our bodies to be more in sync and more productive!

□

Homemade Ingredients

These items are the foundation upon which you can build any number of homemade dishes. Starting from the right ingredients is essential to the Paleo Lifestyle, and sometimes that means preparing your own.

Take some time each week to prepare the items you'll need, and your week will be easy and stress free.

Basic Yellow Mustard

Mustard is a simple condiment that adds to a large number of more complex sauce recipes. It works as an emulsifier, as well as adding a salty flavor to anything you use it in.

Ingredients:

1 1/4 cup ground dry mustard seed
1 cup water
3/4 cup white distilled vinegar
2 tsp tapioca flour
1 tsp sea salt
1/2 tsp turmeric
1/4 tsp garlic powder
1/4 tsp paprika

Directions:

1. In a medium saucepan over medium heat, bring water and vinegar to a boil.

2. Add mustard seed, salt, turmeric, garlic and paprika. Whisk vigorously.

3. Whisk in tapioca flour. Allow to simmer for 5 min, or until mixture has a thick, paste-like texture.

4. Chill at least 2 hours before using. Store in an airtight container. Keeps up to 1 month.

5. Tip: to make whole grain mustard, replace about half of the ground mustard with whole mustard seeds.

Yield: about 2 cups.

Mayonnaise

Homemade mayo is more natural and much tastier than the store bought variety. It is very easy to make and also enables you to build a large catalog of dips, dressings and sauces.

Ingredients:

1 tsp mustard
2 tbsp cider vinegar
1 tbsp fresh-squeezed lemon juice
1 tsp salt
2 egg yolks
1 1/2 cups grapeseed oil

Directions:

1. In a large mixing bowl combine first five ingredients. Using an electric hand mixer or a whisk (if you're a really good whisker!) whip ingredients together until they reach a frothy consistency.

2. Add oil a few drops at a time, whisking constantly. It helps to have a bowl that will stay in place while you are doing this, or to have a helper add the oil. Take your time at first, only add a few drops every few seconds. Once the mixture starts to lighten, you can start adding the oil faster, maybe 2-3 tbsp at a time. Once it reaches a thick, mayo-like consistency, you can add the remaining oil 1/4 cup at a time. When all oil is added, continue to mix for another 1-2 min, just to ensure everything is incorporated and the texture is perfect.

3. Keep in the refrigerator in an airtight container (a mason jar or an old mayo bottle work great) Keeps up to 1 week.

Yield: about 1 1/2 cups.

Ghee (Clarified Butter)

Ghee is a purified butter product that removes all milk solids. It is very simple to make at home, and useful in everything from savory to sweet dishes; especially Paleo baking.

Ingredients:

1-2 lbs butter (depending on how much you want)

Directions:

1. In a medium saucepan over low heat, melt the butter. As soon as it's melted you will see the white milk solids separate from the transparent yellow fat. When the butter begins to boil, this means the water is cooking off. The bubbles will gradually get smaller, until they reach a foam-like consistency. The milk solids will begin to brown and clump together at this point. Once these clumps start falling to the bottom, remove the pan from the heat.

2. Strain the hot butter through a cheesecloth into a heat-safe container (a glass jar works great). Store in the refrigerator as you would butter. Keeps up to 2 months.

Yield: a little less than 2 cups per pound of butter.

Rendered Animal Fat

Animal fat is probably the best cooking fat for the Paleo Lifestyle, at least health-wise.

Some fats will smoke at lower temperatures, so it's not always ideal, but this is a great way to waste less, which is environmentally responsible.

Ingredients:

Trimmings, skin or sinew from any grass-fed, all-natural meat.

*Note: it's not generally a good idea to use more than one kind of meat when rendering animal fat. Some fats will have different chemical properties like smoke point, and will also have different flavors.

Directions:

1. When cooking meats, save any trimmings, unwanted skin and sinew from your meat.

2. Place trimmings, etc. in a large stock pot over low heat and allow to cook, stirring

often, until fat has liquefied. This will take different amounts of time depending on the ingredients, and the amounts you use.

3. When fat begins to boil, this means the water is cooking out. Allow to boil for 15 minutes. You may want to cover the pot with a mesh grease guard, to prevent mess, but DO NOT cover the pot with a lid, as this will prevent the water form escaping.

4. After about 15 minutes, all water should be boiled off, and fat should not be bubbling as aggressively. If it's still making a lit of fuss and noise, let it go until it calms down, but don't let the trimmings burn.

5. Strain mixture through a mesh strainer into a heat-proof container like a glass bowl.

6. Strain mixture again through a cheesecloth into your storage container. A mason jar is ideal.

7. Refrigerate up to 1 week.

Yield: variable.

Beef Stock

Beef stock is a great cooking aid. It delivers flavor in a variety of settings.

Ingredients:

Bones, and trimmings from any cut of beef.
*Note: Use the leftover bones and uneaten meat
from a beef dish for even more flavor.
1 onion, halved
2 stalks celery, roughly chopped
2 cloves garlic (or more, if desired)
1 bay leaf
2-3 pods whole allspice
1 tsp whole coriander seed

Directions:

1. Add all ingredients to a large stock pot. Cover with water.

2. Allow to boil over medium heat for 1 hour. Stock is done when it is deep

brown in color.

3. Strain with a mesh strainer or colander. Store in an airtight container. Keeps up to 1 week in the refrigerator, 3 months when frozen.

Yield: variable, up to 1 gallon.

Chicken Stock

Chicken stock is another great cooking aid. Steaming or boiling vegetables with chicken stock will give them extra flavor while keeping things light.

Ingredients:

Bones, skin, trimmings and uneaten meat of 1 whole chicken
1 onion, halved
2 stalks celery, roughly chopped
2 cloves garlic
1 bay leaf
1 sprig fresh thyme
2-3 leaves fresh sage

Directions:

1. Add all ingredients to a large stock pot. Cover with water.

2. Allow to boil over medium heat for 1 hour. Stock is done when it is mellow gold in color.

3. Strain with a mesh strainer or colander. Store in an airtight container. Keeps up to 1 week in the refrigerator, 3 months when frozen.

Yield: variable, up to 1 gallon.

Almond Milk

Almond milk is great if you don't tolerate dairy, and it can be used in almost every way dairy milk can.

Commercially produced almond milk is full of unhealthy additives, but luckily it is very simple to make at home.

Ingredients:

1 cup raw almonds
2 cups filtered water
Raw, organic honey (optional)

Directions:

1. Place your almonds in a resealable container and cover them with water. Soak at least overnight, up to 2 days. The longer you soak them, the creamier the resulting milk.

2. Drain and thoroughly rinse your

almonds after they are done soaking. Add them to a blender or food processor.

3. Pour in the 2 cups of water and blend for 1 minute. Almond milk should be a slightly brownish off-white color.

4. Strain your almond milk through a cheesecloth into a resealable airtight container (again, mason jars are great for this). Keeps in the refrigerator up to 3 days.

5. If you're using the leftover almond meal, dry it thoroughly by pressing with the cheesecloth, then spread it on a baking sheet in a thin layer and put it in the oven on the lowest setting. Roast with the oven door slightly open for about 10 min, or until almond meal is dry.

Yield: about 2 cups almond milk and 1 cup almond meal.

□

Breakfast Recipes

Sometimes breakfast needs to be more than eggs and meat. We know that.

These recipes will give you an idea of how far you can stretch your creativity to keep breakfasts interesting.

Tapioca Crepes

This may not be a crepe, technically, but you can sure use it the same way. The naturally sweet flavor of tapioca flour brings a familiar note to this dish.

Ingredients:

1 cup tapioca flour
1 1/2 tsp baking powder
½ cup warm water
½ cup almond milk
4 eggs
pinch of salt
Ghee for the pan

Directions:

1. In a medium mixing bowl, whisk together the tapioca, coconut, baking powder, soda and salt.

2. In a large mixing bowl, whisk together the eggs, water and coconut milk.

3. Mix the dry ingredients into the wet.

Whisk vigorously until there are very few lumps. Batter will be runny.

4. In a large heavy bottom skillet, melt the ghee.

5. Spoon about 1/4 cup of the batter into the hot pan at a time. Tilt the pan to spread it evenly. Cook 1-2 min, until the edges curl and the crepe comes loose when the pan is shaken. Flip, and cook an additional 30 seconds to 1 min on the other side. Repeat until all batter is used.

6. Top with warm berries or whipped coconut milk. You can even use these crepes as pasta sheets in a Paleo lasagna.

Yield: 3-4 servings.

Fritatta

Fritatta is a traditional Italian egg dish. It's a great way to re-purpose leftovers, and a fast and easy breakfast that you could make every morning.

Ingredients:

6 eggs
2 tbsp coconut or almond milk
Any meats, cheeses, herbs, vegetables or leftovers you desire. The sky is truly the limit here, things as diverse as sweet potatoes, jalapenos, steak, sausage, mushrooms, squash, Parmesan cheese, pepperoni and olives go surprisingly great in fritatta.

Directions:

1. Preheat the oven to 350 degrees.

2. Preheat an oven-safe pan with a few tablespoons of oil or ghee. Add your fillings and sautee until they reach the desired level of doneness. For leftovers, you'll just want to warm them up a bit.

For fresh vegetables you'll want to cook them until they're soft, or even until they're caramelized. For fresh meats like chicken or pork you'll want to cook them all the way through.

3. In a small mixing bowl, whisk together the eggs and coconut/almond milk. Season with salt and pepper.

4. Pour your eggs over the toppings. If you are using any cheese, add it now. Stir lightly to ensure everything is evenly distributed.

5. Transfer the pan to the oven and bake at 350 for 10-15 minutes, until eggs are firm in the middle.

6. Remove from oven and allow to cool for 5-10 minutes. Invert the pan over a cutting board or serving dish. The fritatta should fall right out.

7. Slice and serve! This dish is also great leftover, cold or hot.

Yield: 2-4 servings.

A Perfect Omelet

A perfect omelet is one of the easiest and hardest things to make. Any professional chef will tell you that cooking skill is often measured by how well you make an omelet. With a little practice, you can swing with the big boys.

Ingredients:

3 eggs
Any fillings you desire; cheeses, meats or vegetables

Directions:

1. Preheat a large skillet.

2. While the skillet heats up, dice your fillings, about 1/4 to 1/2 an inch is perfect.

3. Add 1-2 tbsp of ghee or oil to the pan. Add the fillings (except for the cheese, if using) and sautee until they reach the desired level of doneness. For fresh vegetables you'll want to cook them until they're soft, or even

until they're caramelized. For fresh meats like chicken or pork you'll want to cook them all the way through.

4. Remove the fillings from the pan and set aside. Rinse off the pan, making sure to remove anything that stuck to it. Don't use soap, just a firm-bristled brush.

5. Reheat the clean pan over medium heat for about 2-3 minutes. It is very important that you use only medium heat, high heat will result in a burnt omelet.

6. While the pan reheats, whisk your eggs. You want them as well-blended as you can possibly get them; the better mixed they are, the better texture your omelet will have. An immersion blender is the ideal tool for this, but a food processor or blender will do nicely as well.

7. Add 2 tbsp ghee or oil to the pan. Pour in your eggs.

8. Allow the eggs to cook for a few minutes. This is the most crucial part of the omelet-making process. The egg that is in direct contact with the pan will begin to cook quickly, while there will be a layer of uncooked liquid on top. As your eggs begin

to firm up, push the edges into the center with the edge of a spatula. Do it gently, making sure not to push them further than an inch or so towards the middle. Tilt the pan around to slosh some of the uncooked liquid into the resulting space and repeat, working your way around the entire omelet until almost all of the liquid is cooked.

9. At this point you have two options. One, you can add your toppings and cheese, fold your omelet in half and call it a day. Two, if you prefer firmer, fully-cooked eggs, you can flip the eggs over and cook the other side. Flipping is difficult to pull off, so you'll probably rip a few before you do it just right. A nice, broad spatula helps, and the more done your eggs already are before you flip them, the easier it will be. However, even on medium heat, the eggs might burn.

10. Either way, add your fillings and cheese, fold your omelet and plate it up. If you have a particularly heavy, full omelet, you can invert it onto a plate. If not, a spatula should work fine.

Yield: 1 serving.

Homemade Breakfast Sausage

Store-bought breakfast sausage usually comes packed with nitrates, sugar and other things you don't want. Real breakfast sausage is just spiced ground pork. You can make it at home with a minimum of fuss.

Ingredients:

1 pound ground pork
1 tbsp salt
2 tsp pepper
1 tsp ground sage
1 tsp dried thyme
1/2 tsp ground rosemary
1/2 tsp paprika
1/4 tsp cayenne
1/4 tsp ground cinnamon
1/4 tsp ground nutmeg
2 tsp raw, organic honey (if tolerated)

Directions:

1. In a large mixing bowl, combine all

ingredients. Mix with your hands until everything is just distributed. Do not over work the meat.

2. Shape into patties or links and fry until fully cooked, about 3-5 min per side depending on the size of the patty. Serve with eggs or whatever else you like for breakfast.

3. Store any uncooked sausage in a vacuum-packed container, if possible. If not, store in a zip-top bag with as much air removed as possible. Flavors will develop in the refrigerator.

Yield: 1 pound sausage, about 4-6 servings.

The Best Fruit Salad

Fruit salad isn't complicated. It almost seems silly to have a recipe for it. But this recipe is all about showing you just how far you can take it.

Ingredients:

1 small apple, peeled and diced
1 banana, sliced
1/2 cup pineapple chunks
1/2 cup grapes
1 kiwi, peeled and sliced
1 orange, cut into mandarins (peel it then slice out the sections, discarding the interior skins)
1/2 cup sliced strawberries
1/4 cup blueberries
1/4 cup raspberries
1/2 cup melon cubes (use whatever is the ripest; cantaloupe, honeydew or watermelon)
1 avocado, diced
2 tbsp lime juice
1 tsp salt
1/4 cup raw honey diluted with a few tbsp of warm water (optional)

Directions:

1. Dice all of your ingredients to a similar size. 1/4 to 1/2 inch pieces are ideal for eating with a spoon.

2. Add all fruits to a large mixing bowl. Drizzle with lime juice and sprinkle with salt. If using, add diluted honey.

3. Mix well. Serve by itself, or on top of tapioca crepes.

Yield: 5-6 cups, 2-3 servings

□

Sauces and Marinades

A great sauce or marinade can be the difference between eating the same thing every night, and exploring a world of culinary possibilities.

Here are a few basics to get you started.

Homemade Salsa

You might be able to find store-bought salsa that's Paleo-friendly, but why would you bother when making it fresh is so easy and tastes so much better?

Ingredients:

1 pound fresh tomatoes
1/4 onion
1-2 jalapenos (depending on how hot you want it – use habaneros if you're a fire-eater!)
1/4 cup cilantro
Juice and zest of 1/2 lime
salt and pepper to taste

Directions:

1. Roughly chop all ingredients, just small enough so they will fit in the food processor or blender. *For extra flavor, char the peppers and onions directly over the fire of a gas stove, or by putting them in a 500 degree oven for 5-10 min.

2. Add all ingredients to a food processor or blender and blend until desired consistency is reached. For chunkier salsa, pulse 5-10 times, for thinner salsa, blend 1 minute.

3. Serve over Pollo Asada or with raw vegetables for dipping.

Yield: about 1 quart.

Balsamic Vinaigrette

A basic salad dressing that goes good on any vegetable. Once you start making your own dressings, you'll realize just how many things you can put in them, and you'll never go back to the store-bought stuff.

Ingredients:

1/2 cup balsamic vinegar
1/2 cup olive oil
2 tsp fresh oregano
2 tsp fresh thyme
1 clove garlic, minced
2 tsp black pepper
1 pinch salt

Directions:

1. Combine all ingredients in a food processor and puree until smooth.

2. Serve over spring mix or drizzled over fresh strawberries.

Yield: about 1 cup.

Tomato Basil Marinara

This is about as easy as tomato sauce gets. Forget the long cook times and heavy doses of sugar in traditional recipes; this small, quick rendition is easy enough to make several times a week.

Ingredients:

4 roma or plum tomatoes, quartered
2 tbsp olive oil
1/2 cup beef or chicken stock
1/2 onion, diced
2 cloves garlic, minced
2 tbsp fresh basil, chopped
2 tbsp fresh parsley, chopped
salt and pepper, to taste

Directions:

1. In a large stock pot over medium-high heat, sautee the garlic and onions in olive oil until soft.

2. Add tomatoes and stock, season with salt

and pepper and bring to a simmer.

3. Reduce heat to low, cover, and allow to simmer 30 min, stirring frequently.

4. Stir in remaining ingredients in and transfer to a blender or food processor. Blend until smooth.

5. Serve over shredded, blanched zucchini for a decidedly pasta-like entree.

Yield: about 2 cups.

BBQ Marinade

This marinade is an easy way to create rich BBQ flavor without a smoker, and more importantly without sugar-laden BBQ sauce.

Ingredients:

2 cloves garlic, minced
1/2 onion, diced
1/2 cup, plus 1 tbsp grapeseed oil
1/4 cup all-natural, unsweetened apple juice
1/4 cup apple cider vinegar
1/4 cup coconut aminos
2 tbsp raw, organic honey (optional)
1 tbsp salt
1 tbsp black pepper
1 tbsp paprika
2 tsp ground cumin
2 tsp coriander seed
2 tsp chili powder
2 tsp ground mustard
1 tsp cayenne
1 tsp ground sage
1 tsp celery seed

Directions:

1. In a medium saucepan over high heat, sautee the onion and garlic in the 1 tbsp grapeseed oil

2. When onions are nicely charred, add remaining ingredients. Bring to a simmer, whisking frequently.

3. Pour over meat and marinate at least 4 hours, up to 2 days in refrigerator.

Yield: enough for 2 lbs of meat

Mexican Marinade

This spicy, herbaceous marinade gives you the authentic, south-of-the-border flavor you need. Great over chicken, pork or beef.

Ingredients:

1/2 onion, diced
2 cloves garlic, minced
1 jalapeno, ribs and seeds removed
1/2 cup plus 2 tbsp olive oil
Juice and zest of 1 lime
Juice and zest of 1 orange
1/4 cup fresh cilantro, packed
3 tbsp ground cumin
1 tsp ground coriander seed
1 tsp salt
1 tsp black pepper

Directions:

1. In a small skillet over high heat, sautee the garlic, onion and jalapeno in the 2 tbsp olive oil.

2. While vegetables are sauteing, add remaining ingredients to a food processor or blender.

3. When vegetables are well charred, add to food processor.

4. Blend on high about 1 min, until marinade reaches an even consistency.

5. Pour over meat and marinate at least 4 hours, up to 2 days in the refrigerator. If using on seafood, do not marinate more than 2 hours.

Yield: enough for 2 lbs of meat

Entrees

For Paleo eaters, the distinction between a lunch recipe and a dinner recipe can be a subtle one.

In our opinion, the only real difference is whether or not the dish travels well.

Paleo lunches need to be good reheated, so steak and certain veggie sides might not be great for lunch.

Either way, the recipes here are better categorized as entrees.

Pot Roast With Butternut Squash

Slow cooked beef is one of the tastiest things you can eat. There's something about pot roast that just says home. This recipe calls upon the slightly sweet flavor of butternut squash to replace the traditional white potatoes.

Ingredients:

2 tbsp rendered animal fat
2 lbs beef chuck roast or other beef roast
4 cups beef stock
2 cups butternut squash, cubed
3 carrots, roughly chopped
1 onion, roughly chopped
4 cloves garlic
2 bay leaves
2 sprigs fresh thyme
Salt and pepper, to taste

Directions:

1. Preheat the oven to 350 degrees.

2. In a dutch oven over medium-high heat, melt animal fat. Add onion and garlic,

sautee 3-5 min, until onions are slightly charred.

3. Add beef, brown on both sides, 2-3 min per side.

4. Deglaze pan with beef stock. Add remaining ingredients. Cover and transfer dutch oven to the preheated oven. Cook for 2-3 hours, until beef is fall-apart tender and vegetables are very soft. Serve with broth for dipping.

Yield: 4 servings.

Cajun Roast Chicken

While this might not be a traditional Cajun dish, it's easy to incorporate those rich, spicy flavors into your Paleo Lifestyle.

Ingredients:

1 small chicken, cut into pieces or pre-cut legs, wings and thighs
1 onion, quartered
1 green bell pepper, halved, seeds removed
1 red bell pepper, halved, seeds removed
3-4 stalks celery, cut into large pieces (2-3")
2 tbsp ghee
2 tbsp grapeseed oil
2 tsp salt
1 tbsp black pepper
2 tsp paprika
1 tsp chili powder
2 tsp dried parsley
1/2 tsp celery seed
1/2 tsp cayenne
1/4 tsp chili flake

Directions:

1. Preheat oven to 350 degrees.

2. In a small mixing bowl, stir together all spices until uniform. Rub over chicken until all sides are evenly coated.

3. Heat ghee in a large cast-iron skillet over medium-high heat.

4. Add chicken to pan and sear 6-7 min on one side.

5. In a large mixing bowl, toss the onions, peppers and celery with the grapeseed oil. Season to taste with salt and black pepper, or any remaining spice mixture.

6. Flip chicken pieces. Add vegetables to pan, arranging so that everything is in contact with the bottom of the pan. You don't want any chicken pieces laying on top of veggies, it may cause the veggies to burn

7. Transfer the pan to the oven and roast until chicken reaches an internal temperature of 165 degrees or higher. This may take up to 30 minutes.

8. Serve over riced cauliflower with lemon slices and fresh herbs.

Yield: about 4 servings.

Mustard-Crusted Pork Chops

Ingredients:

1 tbsp whole brown mustard seeds
1 tbsp whole yellow mustard seeds
1 tbsp homemade mustard
1/4 cup almond meal
1/2 cup homemade mayo
salt and black pepper to taste
2 thick-cut pork chops
2 tbsp grapeseed oil

Directions:

1. Preheat the oven to 350 degrees.

2. Heat grapeseed oil in a large, oven safe skillet.

3. Season the pork chops with salt and pepper. Place them in the pan and sear on one side for 2-3 min, until lightly browned.

4. Flip and transfer to oven. Bake at 350 until pork reaches an internal temperature of 145

degrees, about 10 minutes.

5. Remove pork from oven. Heat the broiler to its highest setting, or raise the oven to 500 degrees.

6. In a small mixing bowl, combine mustard, mustard seeds, mayo, almond meal and black pepper. Spread over pork with a butter knife.

7. Broil or bake the pork for 2-3 min, until crust begins to caramelize.

8. Serve with sauteed greens or parsnip puree.

Yield: 2 servings.

Perfect Steak

The perfect steak to fit your taste is all about picking the right cut, and cooking it to its ideal temperature. Preferences may very, but there's a steak out there for everybody.

Ingredients:

Your choice of steak:

1. If you like a rich, fatty flavor and don't mind a little gristle, go with a ribeye.
2. For a leaner but still tender and juicy cut, filet is the best option.
3. New York Strip is a nice, middle-of-the-road option.
4. Sirloin is one of the more inexpensive cuts, but requires a little marination to really make it pop.

salt and pepper to taste
garlic powder (optional)

Directions:

1. Buy fresh steak. If you freeze it, make sure to do so in a vacuum-sealed bag immediately after purchase. If you freeze your steak before eating it, allow it to thaw at room temperature for 2 hours, or until completely thawed.

2. Season your steak on both sides with salt and pepper, and garlic powder if desired. Other great additions include paprika, mustard seeds, or freshly chopped herbs.

3. Allow the steak to rest at room temperature for 30 minutes. The salt will tenderize the steak and carry all the other flavors into the meat.

4. Grill your steak over high heat on a grill, flat-top or cast iron skillet. There are many ways to check the doneness of a steak, but the most reliable is temperature. Use the following list:
    125 degrees................rare
    130-135 degrees.........medium rare
    135-140 degrees.........medium
    140-150 degrees.........medium well
    150 degrees and up.....well done

5. For fattier cuts like ribeye or strip,

medium rare to medium is recommended. Sirloins are best marinated and served medium to well. Filet may be served very rare, and is still quite tender and flavorful when well done.

6. When your steak is at your desired temperature, remove it from the heat and allow it to rest for 10 minutes. This allows the juices to be locked in. If you cut your steak without resting it, the juices will run out and you will have a flavorless, dry steak.

7. Serve with cauliflower puree and steamed green beans for a hearty, homey meal.

Yield: 1-2 servings.

Chipotle-Lime Fish Tacos

Fish tacos are a healthy meal that everybody loves. Simply substituting the tortillas for a sturdy lettuce like butter or Boston bring them into the Paleo fold.

Ingredients:

4 filets wild-caught whitefish (cod, pollock, or mahi-mahi work well)
1/4 cup grapeseed oil, plus more for the grill
2 tsp chipotle chili powder
salt and black pepper, to taste
8 large leaves butter or iceberg lettuce
1/2 cup homemade salsa
1 avocado, diced
lime juice, to garnish
1/4 cup fresh cilantro, chopped
1/2 cup cabbage, shredded
1/4 cup coconut milk

Directions:

1. Preheat the grill to high heat and oil the grill grate with grapeseed oil.

2. Toss the shredded cabbage and cilantro with the coconut milk, some of the lime juice and a little black pepper. Set aside.

3. Gently rub your fish filets with olive oil and season lightly with salt, pepper, and chipotle chili powder.

4. Grill the fish 3-4 min on each side, flipping only when the fish is ready to release. If you stick a spatula under it and the fish doesn't want to come up, leave it alone. Check again in 30-45 seconds.

5. When your fish filets are done, remove them from the heat and cut each one in half lengthwise.

6. Arrange the fish on the lettuce leaves. Top with a small drizzle of salsa, a few cubes of avocado, a little of the cabbage mixture, and a spritz of lime juice. Wrap and enjoy!

Yield: 8 tacos, about 2-4 servings.

Side Dishes

Mixing and matching sides is a great way to keep variety in your diet. Accordingly, we've kept the sides out of the entree recipes for the most part, and presented them here so you can find the pairings that work best for your individual tastes.

Coleslaw

Traditional coleslaw relies on heaping cups of sugar to deliver that sweet and salty bite. The Paleo rendition employs the natural sweetness of coconut milk, with an optional touch of honey.

Ingredients:

4 cups cabbage, green, red, or both, shredded
1 cup carrots, shredded
1/4 cup fresh parsley, chopped
1/2 cup homemade mayo
1/3 cup coconut milk
1/2 tsp ground coriander
salt and black pepper to taste
2 tsp raw, organic honey (optional)

Directions:

1. For finer slaw, shred your cabbage and carrots using a cheese grater or the shredding attachment of a food processor. For rougher slaw, cut cabbage with a knife.

2. Add all ingredients to a large mixing bowl and stir until everything is well blended. Refrigerate until ready to serve.

3. Serve with BBQ marinated meats or seasoned fish.

Yield: about 5 cups.

Green Bean Grill Pack

The foil grill pack is one of the best ways to prepare your veggies when cooking out, and this method delivers a rich and flavorful side that goes great with everything.

Ingredients:

4 cups of fresh green beans, trimmed.
1/2 onion
4 strips uncured bacon
1/4 cup grapeseed oil
salt and pepper, to taste

Directions:

1. Lay out a very large sheet of broad foil on the counter. 18" x 24" is ideal.

2. Take the 1/2 onion and cut it in half again. Separate the layers and lay half of them on the foil. Season with salt and pepper and drizzle with oil.

3. Cut the bacon strips in half. Lay half of

them over the onions. Season with salt
and pepper.

4. Add the green beans to a large mixing
   bowl. Season heavily with salt and
   pepper and drizzle with olive oil. Place
   them atop the bacon and form into a
   rough rectangle.

5. Top with more bacon, season with more
   salt and pepper.

6. Top with more onions, season with more
   salt and pepper and a final drizzle of oil.

7. Fold two edges of the foil together and
   roll tight. Crimp in the sides to make a
   little pillow.

8. Preheat the grill to high heat.

9. Grill the foil package for 20 min on each
   side. Onions will be charred, bacon will
   be almost crisp and green beans will be
   nicely steamed. Serve with steaks for
   the perfect paleo meal.

Yield: about 4 servings.

Broccoli Salad

Broccoli salad is a great accompaniment to a variety of dishes. It adds a cooling bite to spicy meats, and mixed with simply grilled chicken makes a great sack lunch.

Ingredients:

2 cups broccoli crowns, finely diced
1/4 cup slivered almonds
2 tbsp onion, minced
4 strips uncured bacon, cooked and crumbled
1/2 cup paleo mayo
salt and pepper to taste
1/4 cup shredded cheddar (optional)

Directions:

1. Add all ingredients to a medium mixing bowl and stir until everything is evenly distributed.

2. Serve with cold grilled chicken or alongside a cup of hot soup.

Yield: 2-3 servings.

Parsnip and Carrot Latkes

This delicious fried side is great at breakfast, lunch or dinner. Hot or cold, plain or served with a little home made mayo and mustard, these crispy veggie cakes are going to make you wonder why people ever started cultivating potatoes in the first place.

Ingredients:

2 cups parsnips, shredded
2 cups carrots, shredded
2 tbsp fresh parsley, chopped
1 tsp fresh thyme, chopped
2 eggs, beaten
salt and pepper to taste
coconut oil, for frying

Directions:

1. Heat coconut oil in a large cast iron skillet over medium-high heat. Use enough so that the melted oil comes up about 1/4 to 1/2 an inch from the bottom of the pan.

2. In a large mixing bowl, stir together all other ingredients until well incorporated.

3. Working in batches, form the vegetable mixture into patties in your hands. Lay them gently in the hot oil, being careful not to splash or burn yourself.

4. Fry in one side until golden brown, about 5 min, then flip. Fry the other side until golden brown.

5. Remove from oil and place on paper towels to drain. Season with more salt immediately after removing the patties from the oil.

6. Serve with poached eggs or alongside a Paleo meatloaf.

Yield: about 4-6 servings.

Grilled Salad

As odd as this might sound, grilled salad is one of the most unique dishes you will ever make, and it is also one of the easiest. You will wow your guests with this one.

Ingredients:

2-4 heads of sturdy lettuce (romaine is the best, but iceberg, green leaf and red leaf also work)
grapeseed oil, to coat
salt and pepper, to taste
4-6 tbsp salad dressing of choice

Directions:

1. Peel the wilted outer leaves off the lettuce. Cut each head in half, *leaving the stem in.* You need the stem to keep the lettuce together while it's on the grill.

2. Season to taste with oil, salt and pepper, making sure to coat all sides and as many of the inner leaves as you can get to without ripping the heads apart.

3. Preheat the grill to high heat.

4. Grill the heads for 1-2 minutes on each side. You want some light charring of the outer leaves. Err on the side of undercooking, otherwise you will have a completely wilted salad. Some wilting is to be expected, but too much makes this dish greasy and unsatisfying.

5. Remove your lettuce heads from the grill and chop them as you would for a fresh salad.

6. Toss with the dressing of your choice, but don't use too much, as the lettuce is already seasoned.

7. Serve with grilled steaks or pork chops.

Yield: 2-4 servings.

Dessert Recipes

At first, it might seem like real desserts are impossible with the Paleo Lifestyle. Nothing could be further from the truth. Paleo Desserts are every bit as rich and satisfying as traditional desserts, only they won't leave you feeling bogged down in a blood sugar trench.

Some of these recipes will use ingredients that your Paleo Lifestyle may not tolerate.

Removing things like honey or dark chocolate will result in a less decadent dessert, but still better than using your 20% on something you'll regret.

Chocolate-Dipped Almond Cookies

These little delights are a quick and satisfying sweet snack that you can grab when you have a craving. If you don't tolerate honey or dark chocolate, they still make a surprisingly satisfying bite.

Ingredients:

1/2 pound almond meal
1 egg
1 tbsp ghee, melted
1 tsp baking powder
1 tbsp raw, organic honey
1/4 tsp cinnamon
1/8 tsp nutmeg
1/8 tsp allspice
pinch salt
6-8 oz dark chocolate (about 2 bars)

Directions:

1. Preheat the oven to 350 degrees.

2. In a food processor, pulse together the almond meal, eggs, ghee, baking powder,

honey, cinnamon, nutmeg and allspice until a dough forms.

3. Place the dough between two sheets of parchment and roll flat with a rolling pin. Remove the top sheet of parchment. Quickly and carefully invert the cookies onto a well-greased sheet pan. Cut into squares using a pizza cutter or a knife.

4. Bake at 350 degrees for 12-14 minutes. Remove your cookies from the oven and allow to cool completely.

5. Make a double boiler by positioning a glass mixing bowl atop a saucepan filled with about 1" of boiling water. Add the chocolate and whisk until smooth. Extra dark chocolate will take longer to melt than milk chocolate.

6. Dip each of the cooled cookies halfway in the chocolate. Place on a fresh sheet of parchment and allow to cool at room temperature until chocolate is firm. This may take up to 2 hours.

Yield: about 20 cookies

Almond Crust Berry Tart

Using a crust recipe similar to the almond cookies, this delicious dinner party dessert is sure to satisfy even non-Paleo guests while keeping your conscience clean.

Ingredients:

1 lb almond flour
2 large eggs
2 tbsp ghee, melted
1 tsp salt
1/4 tsp ground nutmeg
1/4 tsp ground cinnamon
1 cup blackberries
1 cup blueberries
1 cup strawberries
1/4 cup raw, organic honey

Directions:

1. In a large food processor, pulse together almond flour, salt, nutmeg and cinnamon.

2. Add eggs and butter and pulse until a
    dough forms.

3. Press dough into a greased 9-inch pie
    pan with your hands. Bake at 350° until
    golden brown, about 15 minutes.
    Remove crust from oven and allow to
    cool.

4. In a medium mixing bowl, combine
    berries and honey.

5. Pour the filling into the crust. Return
    tart to oven for 10 min. Allow to cool to
    room temperature before serving.

Yield: about 8 servings.

Creamy Coconut Popsicles

These creamy frozen treats are the perfect thing to feed the kids on a hot summer's afternoon. If you don't have a popsicle mold, make them in an ice cube tray for a poppable snack.

Ingredients:

3 cups coconut milk
1 cup unsweetened shredded coconut
2 tbsp raw, organic honey

Directions:

1. In a large mixing bowl, whisk together all ingredients until well combined.

2. Pour mixture into a popsicle mold or an ice cube tray. Freeze until completely solid, about 2-3 hours.

3. Serve by the pool on a hot day.

Yield: 6-8 servings

Crispy Fruit Parfait

This delectable recipe uses a neat trick to imitate whipped cream. Once you've tried it, you'll be using it on all sorts of things.

Ingredients:

2 cans full-fat coconut milk, refrigerated
2 tbsp raw, organic honey, divided
1/2 cup almond meal
1/2 cup sliced strawberries
1/4 cup raspberries
1/4 cup blueberries

Directions:

1. Refrigerate the coconut milk overnight. This will cause the milk to separate from the cream. The milk will settle to the bottom, while the cream will settle on top.

2. Open the can from the bottom and pour out the coconut milk. Save for use in other

recipes.

3. Scrape the coconut cream into a large mixing bowl. Add 1 tbsp honey and whip with an electric hand mixer until light and fluffy.

4. Preheat oven to 350 degrees.

5. In a separate mixing bowl, stir the remaining tbsp of honey into the almond meal. Spread mixture onto a parchment-lined cookie sheet and bake at 350 for 5-10 min, until lightly browned. Scrape off of the parchment and set aside.

6. In a serving dish or glass, layer each parfait as follows: coconut cream, almond meal, berries, almond meal, coconut cream berries, coconut cream and top with any remaining almond meal.

7. Serve as a dessert or a sweet breakfast.

Yield: 2 servings.

Apple Crisp

You might not be able to make traditional apple pie, but you can sure get close with this warm, delicious apple crisp!

Ingredients:

2 cups almond flour
1/2 tsp salt
1 tsp ground cinnamon
1/2 tsp ground nutmeg
1/2 cup ghee, melted
1/4 cup honey
1/2 tsp vanilla extract
5 medium apples, peeled, cored and sliced

Directions:

1. Preheat the oven to 350 degrees

2. In a large mixing bowl, combine almond flour, salt, cinnamon and nutmeg, butter, honey, and vanilla. Mix until well combined.

3. Arrange apples to cover a medium baking dish. Sprinkle topping over apples and cover with foil. Bake at 350 for 50 min.

4. Remove foil and bake an additional 10 min.

5. Serve piping hot with a dollop of whipped coconut cream!

Yield: 4-6 servings.

Snack Recipes

Paleo snacks require a little more prep time than, say, opening a bag of chips, but the tradeoff is that you will be able to munch guilt-free, without feeling deprived of anything. Prepping snacks for the week is something to fill a few hours on a Sunday, and it will save you a boatload of time during your busy week.

"CauliCorn"

If you have a hard time sitting down to a movie without a bowl of popcorn, this little trick will give you that satisfying crunch and buttery flavor you crave.

Ingredients:

1 head cauliflower, chopped
1 quart of grapeseed oil, for frying
2 tbsp ghee, melted
salt, to taste

Directions:

1. Cut the cauliflower so that you remove as much of the stems as possible. You want to end up with popcorn-sized crowns that you can eat by the handful, just like the real thing.

2. Heat the oil in a large cast iron skillet over medium-high heat. Fill the skillet so that there is about an inch of oil in it.

3. Carefully drop the cauliflower crowns into the hot oil. You may need to work in batches; you don't want to crowd the pan. Pieces should not be piling up on top of each other.

4. Fry the cauliflower until it is crispy and slightly caramelized, about 5-8 min. Remove from oil and drain over paper towels.

5. Transfer drained cauliflower into a serving bowl.

6. Melt the ghee in the microwave. Drizzle over the cauliflower and season with salt.

7. Turn off the lights and hit play!

Yield: about 4 servings.

Beef Jerky

Even without a dehydrator, you can make great beef jerky at home. All it takes is a little patience and the right cut of meat.

Ingredients:

2 pounds of *very* lean beef (top round is good, or well-trimmed flank steak. Fat will go rancid in storage, so you want it as lean as possible)
1/2 cup coconut aminos
1 tbsp black pepper
1 tsp salt
1 tsp garlic powder
1 tsp onion powder
1 tsp crushed red pepper (optional)

Directions:

1. Preheat the oven to the lowest setting.

2. Place thawed beef in the freezer for 30 min to help firm it up.

3. Slice beef into 1/4" thick strips. If you prefer jerky that is easier to chew, cut against the grain, or diagonally. If you prefer your jerky very tough, cut along the grain. Make sure to trim away *all* fat.

4. Place beef in a glass baking dish and cover with the remaining ingredients. Stir to make sure everything is well coated. Refrigerate uncovered at least overnight, up to 24 hours.

5. Arrange strips of beef on a wire rack above a baking sheet with raised sides. Bake at your oven's lowest setting with the door partially opened. Check periodically; meat may take up to 4 hours to dry completely. Store in a zip-top bag for up to 2 months.

Yield: 10-12 oz.

Dried Balsamic Strawberries

Dried strawberries are nature's licorice. They don't take too long to make, and they're incredibly easy. Try them as a snack, or even on a salad!

Ingredients:

2 cups strawberries, halved or quartered
balsamic vinegar, for drizzling
grapeseed oil, for the cookie sheet

Directions:

1. Preheat the oven to the lowest setting.

2. Lightly grease a cookie sheet with oil. This will ensure your strawberries don't stick.

3. Arrange the strawberries on the cookie sheet and drizzle lightly with balsamic vinegar. Place in the oven and bake with the oven door slightly open for about 40-50 min, until berries are completely dry.

4. Store in an airtight container for up to a
    week (though you'll probably finish them
    long before that!)

Yield: about 1 cup.

Paleo Hummus

The chickpea is a legume, so it's definitely out of your Paleo Lifestyle. But the cashew is a Paleo-friendly tree nut, and works just as well in this traditional Middle Eastern dip. Tahini is made from sesame seeds, which are okay for Paleo people, so long as you're not having them in large quantities every day.

Ingredients:

    1 cup raw cashews
    1/4 cup tahini
    3 cloves garlic
    Juice of 1 lemon
    1 tbsp olive oil, plus more for drizzling
    1 tsp salt
    1/2 tsp cumin
    1/4 cup almond milk

Directions:

1. Place cashews in a resealable container and cover with water. Soak overnight in the refrigerator.

2. Drain cashews and rinse thoroughly.

3. Place cashews, tahini and garlic cloves in a food processor and blend until it reaches a thick, paste-like consistency.

4. Add lemon juice, olive oil, salt and cumin. Blend until well incorporated.

5. Add coconut milk 1 tbsp at a time until desired texture is reached. For thinner hummus, more may be required.

6. Top with a drizzle of olive oil and a sprinkle of paprika if desired.

Yield: about 1½ cups.

Trail Mix

Trail mix has to be one of the oldest snacks out there. It's so simple to make, and so obviously great. We hope this little recipe keeps you full and energized on your next outdoor adventure.

Ingredients:

1/2 cup roasted cashews
1/2 cup roasted almonds
1/2 cup roasted pecans
1/4 cup sunflower kernels
1/4 cup roasted pumpkin seeds
1/2 cup dried strawberries, diced
1/2 cup dried blueberries
1/2 cup dried apples, diced
1/2 cup dark chocolate, chopped
salt, to taste

Directions:

1. If you prefer buying raw nuts, roast your own nuts in the oven at 350 degrees for about 12-15 minutes, stirring once or twice

during cooking.

2. Dry the blueberries and apples using the same method as the strawberries. Blueberries won't take as long, about 30 min. Apples will take a little longer, up to an hour. Watch both carefully.

3. Once your ingredients are prepared to your liking, all you have to do is toss them all in a zip-top bag and shake them up. Grab a handful of the way out the door, or pack little baggies up for the kid's lunch.

Yield: 4 cups.

BONUS RECIPES

Here are a few extra recipes for you to try! Some of these are a touch more complicated, but still easy enough for beginners!

Tuna Tartare

Tuna Tartare is an incredible way to eat fresh fish. If the idea of raw fish turns you off, this dish might just change your mind.

Ingredients:

1 pound fresh (never frozen) tuna steak
1/4 cup olive oil
Juice and zest of 1 lime
1 tsp fresh grated horseradish
1 tsp mustard
1 tbsp coconut aminos
1 tsp crushed red pepper
2 tsp salt
1 tsp pepper
2 green onions, minced
1/2 jalapeno, ribs and seeds removed, diced
1 avocado, diced
2 tsp toasted sesame seeds
thinly sliced cucumber for dipping

Directions:

1. Dice the tuna steak into 1/4" cubes and place in a medium mixing bowl.

2. In a separate mixing bowl, whisk together oil, lime juice, lime zest, horseradish, mustard, coconut aminos, crushed red pepper, salt and pepper.

3. Pour sauce over tuna. Add green onions, jalapeno and sesame seeds. Mix well.

4. Add the avocado and gently fold it in, making sure not to crush it into guacamole.

5. Allow the tartare to chill in the refrigerator for 1 hour before serving. Serve with sliced cucumbers for dipping.

Yield: 5-6 servings.

Ceviche

Ceviche is a traditional appetizer in many Latin cultures. It is a rich, acid-cooked seafood salad often made with tomatoes. If you liked the tuna tartare, you're going to love this!

Ingredients:

7-10 oz fresh (never frozen) whitefish (cod, pollock, etc)
6-8 oz medium shrimp, peeled, tail off, cooked and chilled
juice of 1 lime
juice of 1 lemon
1 medium tomato, diced
1/4 onion, minced
1 jalapeno, ribs and seeds removed, diced
2 tbsp fresh cilantro, chopped
1 avocado, diced
salt and pepper to taste

Directions:

1. Dice the whitefish into 1/4 to 1/2 inch cubes. Place in a medium mixing bowl and toss

with lime and lemon juice. Cover and refrigerate 15-20 min, until fish is white throughout.

2. Add all remaining ingredients, except for the avocado. Toss until well mixed.

3. Transfer to a serving dish and top with avocado. Serve with sliced cucumbers and celery for dipping, or just eat with a fork!

Yield: 4-5 servings.

Sausage and Egg Muffin Cups

These little beauties are a great grab-and-go breakfast. Just form them up the night before, crack the eggs in the morning, bake for 15 minutes and you're off!

Ingredients:

8 oz homemade breakfast sausage
1/4 onion, diced
1/2 red bell pepper, diced
1 tbsp grapeseed oil
2/3 cup cheese, shredded (optional)
6 eggs

Directions:

1. Consult the previous chapter for a great sausage recipe, or just use plain ground pork.

2. Press the raw sausage into the cups of a muffin tin so that you have a "crust" of

sausage. You should have enough to cover 6 cups.

3. In a medium skillet, heat the grapeseed oil over high heat. Add the pepper and onion and sautee about 5-8 min, until soft and slightly caramelized.

4. Spoon a small amount of the peppers and onions into each sausage cup. Do not fill the cups all the way, only about 1/3 to 1/2 the way up. Discard any extra.

5. Top with a small amount of cheese, if using.

6. If preparing ahead, cover and refrigerate overnight. If not, skip to the next step.

7. Preheat the oven to 350 degrees.

8. Press the peppers and cheese down into the cup lightly, making sure they are all still slightly concave. Crack one egg into each cup and allow it to settle over the center as best you can.

9. Bake at 350 for 15 minutes, until all eggs are set. Rotate once during cooking to ensure eggs cook evenly.

10. Cups should slide out of the tin easily. Put a

few in a resealable container and eat them in the car on the way to work!

Yield: 6 muffins, 2-3 servings.

Classic Ratatouille

This dish doesn't need much fooling around with to make it Paleo. It's all about fresh, natural vegetables cooked simply so their innate flavors can shine through.

Ingredients:

1 large eggplant
2 medium zucchini
1 onion
1 red bell pepper
1 green bell pepper
4 roma tomatoes
2 cloves garlic, minced
1/4 cup grapeseed oil
3 tbsp fresh parsley, chopped
salt and black pepper, to taste

Directions:

1. Preheat the oven to 350 degrees.

2. Slice all the vegetable about 1/4 of an inch thick. Seed the peppers and cut them into

rings.

3. In a large mixing bowl, toss the vegetable in the oil. Add garlic, salt and pepper, and toss until everything is evenly coated.

4. In a large, deep baking dish, layer the vegetables. Ideally, you want them in patterned rows to make a beautiful presentation. Lay each slice diagonally on top of the last, using the vegetables in the same order until you run out.

5. Cover with foil and bake at 350 for 25 minutes. Remove foil and bake an additional 5 minutes, to allow the juices to evaporate.

6. Serve with braised meat or roasted chicken for a traditional continental meal.

Yield: about 6 servings.

Strawberry Almond Muffins

Here's a baked treat that will go great on any holiday table!

Ingredients:

2 cups almond meal
1/2 tsp salt
1/2 tsp baking powder
1 tsp ground cinnamon
1/4 tsp ground nutmeg
1/4 tsp ground allspice
3 eggs
1/2 cup ghee, melted
1/3 cup raw, organic honey
1 cup sliced strawberries
1/4 cup raw, organic honey
1 tsp lemon juice

Directions:

1.   Preheat oven to 350 degrees and grease a

muffin tin.

2. In a large mixing bowl, combine almond meal, salt, baking powder and spices. Mix well.

3. In a separate bowl, whisk together eggs, ghee and honey until smooth.

4. Add wet ingredients to dry and stir until a batter forms.

5. In another small mixing bowl, toss the strawberries with the honey and lemon juice until well coated.

6. Arrange strawberry mixture into the bottom of six of the muffin cups. Pour batter over strawberry mixture. Discard any extra.

7. Bake at 350 for 25-30 minutes, until tops are golden brown. Allow to cool 10-15 min after removing from oven.

8. Invert onto a serving dish and serve as upside-down muffins!

Yield: 6 muffins.

Go! Go! Paleo!

So there we have it. Everything you need to start and enjoy your Paleo journey. Buk and Wanda would be proud of you!

Enjoy the recipes, and don't forget to check out our other fabulous Paleo recipe book, 'Paleo Comfort Foods Cookbook: Super Quick & Easy, Gluten-Free Paleo Comfort Food Recipes'.

Now go tuck in!

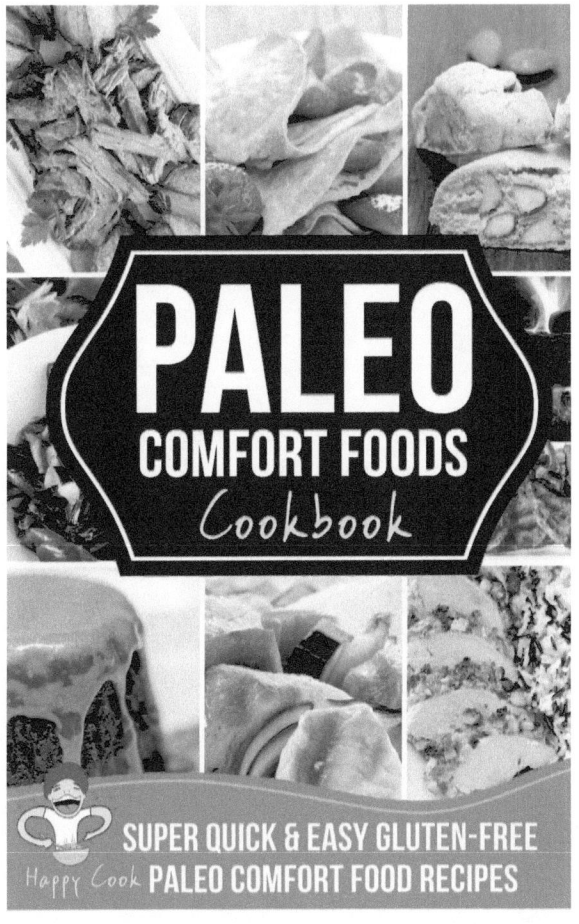

**101 delicious recipes for you to try.
Some you will be familiar with, others
will be lip-smacking new!**